Cambridge Elements ≡

Elements in Emergency Neurosurgery
edited by
Nihal Gurusinghe
Lancashire Teaching Hospital NHS Trust
Peter Hutchinson
University of Cambridge, Society of British Neurological Surgeons, and Royal College of Surgeons of England
Ioannis Fouyas
Royal College of Surgeons of Edinburgh
Naomi Slator
North Bristol NHS Trust
Ian Kamaly-Asl
Royal Manchester Children's Hospital
Peter Whitfield
University Hospitals Plymouth NHS Trust

SPONTANEOUS INTRACRANIAL HAEMORRHAGE CAUSED BY A NON-ANEURYSMAL BRAIN VASCULAR MALFORMATION

Sherif R. W. Kirollos
The National Hospital for Neurology and Neurosurgery (NHNN)

Ramez W. Kirollos
National Neuroscience Institute (NNI)

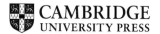

CAMBRIDGE
UNIVERSITY PRESS

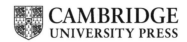

Shaftesbury Road, Cambridge CB2 8EA, United Kingdom

One Liberty Plaza, 20th Floor, New York, NY 10006, USA

477 Williamstown Road, Port Melbourne, VIC 3207, Australia

314–321, 3rd Floor, Plot 3, Splendor Forum, Jasola District Centre,
New Delhi – 110025, India

103 Penang Road, #05–06/07, Visioncrest Commercial, Singapore 238467

Cambridge University Press is part of Cambridge University Press & Assessment,
a department of the University of Cambridge.

We share the University's mission to contribute to society through the pursuit of
education, learning and research at the highest international levels of excellence.

www.cambridge.org
Information on this title: www.cambridge.org/9781009439374

DOI: 10.1017/9781009439367

First published 2025

A catalogue record for this publication is available from the British Library

ISBN 978-1-009-43937-4 Paperback
ISSN 2755-0656 (online)
ISSN 2755-0648 (print)

Cambridge University Press & Assessment has no responsibility for the persistence
or accuracy of URLs for external or third-party internet websites referred to in this
publication and does not guarantee that any content on such websites is, or will
remain, accurate or appropriate.

Every effort has been made in preparing this Element to provide accurate and up-to-
date information which is in accord with accepted standards and practice at the time
of publication. Although case histories are drawn from actual cases, every effort has
been made to disguise the identities of the individuals involved. Nevertheless, the
authors, editors and publishers can make no warranties that the information
contained herein is totally free from error, not least because clinical standards are
constantly changing through research and regulation. The authors, editors and
publishers therefore disclaim all liability for direct or consequential damages resulting
from the use of material contained in this Element. Readers are strongly advised to pay
careful attention to information provided by the manufacturer of any drugs or
equipment that they plan to use.

Spontaneous Intracranial Haemorrhage Caused by a Non-aneurysmal Brain Vascular Malformation

Elements in Emergency Neurosurgery

DOI: 10.1017/9781009439367
First published online: January 2025

Sherif R. W. Kirollos
The National Hospital for Neurology and Neurosurgery (NHNN)

Ramez W. Kirollos
National Neuroscience Institute (NNI)

Author for correspondence: Sherif R. W. Kirollos, sherifkirollos@googlemail.com

Abstract: Emergency management of intracranial haemorrhage due to AVMs, DAVFs, and cavernomas involves addressing both the haemorrhage consequences and the underlying vascular lesion. Clinical evaluation and diagnostic workup identify factors necessitating urgent intervention and define the vascular lesion. Urgent intervention may involve ICH management with increased ICP or CSF drainage for acute hydrocephalus. Definitive intervention for the vascular lesion may coincide with or follow evacuation of the intracranial haematoma. Careful considerations and precautions are taken independently or concurrently with the vascular lesion. Indications and timing for AVM intervention involve determining the bleeding source, evaluating mass effect, and assessing the utility of existing ICHs for microsurgical AVM resection. Modified microsurgical techniques ensure safety. Intervention for DAVF with ICHs or ASDH requires urgent endovascular treatment and surgical nuances. Cavernoma intervention follows straightforward indications and timing, while brainstem cavernomas require careful consideration of early intervention. Aftercare and a team approach are vital.

Keywords: intracerebral haematoma, arteriovenous malformation, dural arteriovenous fistula, cavernoma, decompressive craniectomy

ISBNs: 9781009439374 (PB), 9781009439367 (OC)
ISSNs: 2755-0656 (online), 2755-0648 (print)

Contents

Introduction

Intracerebral haematomas (ICHs) are by far the most common form of spontaneous intracranial haemorrhage. These can extend with associated acute subdural haematomas (ASDHs) or intraventricular haemorrhage (IVH) while spontaneous pure subdural haematomas (SDHs) and IVHs without an ICH are less commonly seen. The common causes of spontaneous ICH are hypertension, amyloid angiopathy, coagulopathy or anticoagulant use, vascular tumours, and other rare causes.[1] Vascular lesions (VLs) resulting in such ICHs include aneurysms, arterio-venous malformations (AVMs), intracranial dural arterio-venous fistulas (DAVFs), and cavernomas.

This Element will discuss emergency management of intracranial haemorrhage secondary to AVMs, DAVFs, and cavernomas. The management of these cases, even in the emergency setting, requires a team approach engaging neurosurgeons and the interventional radiologists. This involves selection of the best management approach as well as complimentary treatment adopted between both approaches that is needed in a number of cases.

Step 1: Evaluation and Workup

When managing a patient with a spontaneous intracranial haemorrhage due to a vascular abnormality, one could be faced with one of three different situations: (1) patients already known to harbour an untreated vascular anomaly that has then bled; (2) those with a highly suspicious radiological appearance of a possible associated underlying VL; and (3) those in whom the radiological distribution and configuration of the haemorrhage warrants further workup to rule out an underlying structural vascular anomaly. There is no consensus on the extent of investigation in many cases: for example, whether to proceed to vascular imaging including digital subtraction angiogram (DSA) in young patients with history of hypertension and an ICH in a 'typical' location for hypertensive haematomas remains a highly variable clinical practice.[1]

Clinical evaluation and diagnostic workup aim to:

(1) identify the factors dictating the need for urgent intervention for the haematoma
(2) establish and define the underlying VL.

Clinical Evaluation

Age, frailty, onset of symptoms, rate of deterioration, and clinical severity influence decision-making and are detailed in the sections on intervention. Age, frailty, and comorbidities not only dictate the appropriateness of invasive intervention, but also whether or not to proceed to complex diagnostic modalities to further evaluate the VL. The history may reveal the suspicion or presence of a known underlying lesion. A history of epilepsy and a family history may be relevant. Assessment of the Glasgow coma scale (GCS) with emphasis on the motor response and identification of relevant neurological deficit, including pupillary abnormalities, should be completed prior to any intubation, if needed.

Investigations

General

These investigations (bloods, electrocardiogram, chest X-ray) are to assess additional aggravating factors and identify fitness for anaesthesia and surgery. Initial assessments and investigation should identify any history of hypertension, diabetes, coagulopathy, or metabolic or electrolyte disturbances.

Imaging

Evaluation of Intracranial Haemorrhage

The types of acute spontaneous intracranial haemorrhage are subdural, subarachnoid haemorrhage (SAH), intraventricular, and parenchymal. The location of haemorrhage aids in establishing the need for further evaluation of possible underlying lesions. However, in emergency situations an important requirement is to establish whether the mass effect of a haemorrhage, or any associated hydrocephalus, requires urgent intervention.

Methods of estimating the size ranging from measuring the largest diameter to sophisticated volumetric calculations exist. Many recommendations for intervention are based on these. However, what is especially important is evaluation of the consequences of this mass effect that takes account of surrounding swelling or, on the contrary, the degree of pre-existing brain atrophy. An example is the degree of fourth ventricular or brainstem compression with cerebellar ICH rather than the size per se.

Evaluation of the Underlying VL in the Emergency Setting

Arterio-venous Malformations

Arterio-venous malformations are characterised by arterio-venous (A-V) shunting via a nidus.[2] They present with intracranial haemorrhage, which is mostly intraparenchymal in 50–60%. A computed tomography (CT) angiogram (CTA) or magnetic resonance image (MRI) will indicate the presence of an AVM and identify the relationship between the nidus and the haematoma, but for planning intervention, a DSA is essential. There are some recent technological advances to establish the role of such techniques, such as dynamic CTA, in planning these procedures. Differentiating an AVM from a DAVF is mandatory.

Dural Arterio-venous Fistulas

The A-V fistula in a DAVF involves dural arterial supply to dural venous channels within leaflets of dura, often without an identifiable nidus.[3] A DSA, including the external carotid injection, is essential. Assessment of associated dural venous sinus anatomy is also important for planning transvenous embolisation should endovascular intervention be considered. However, for surgical consideration, the exact localisation of the cortical venous reflux (CVR) is crucial. Particular attention is needed, as in some cases there are multiple sites of DAVF.

Cavernomas

Cavernomas are abnormally enlarged vascular cavities without intervening parenchyma. The structure of cavernomas is described as tightly packed single-layer endothelial-lined caverns with no tight junctions and surrounding haemosiderin deposition with a wall of organised collagen and a muscular layer. Up to 50% of cases are associated with a developmental venous anomaly (DVA), although this is much less common in familial cases, indicating a possible different pathogenesis.[4]

Cavernomas can be suspected on a CT scan as an area of hyperdensity, but a T2-weighted MRI showing a haemosiderin ring is most helpful. Gradient echo (GE) and susceptibility weighted imaging (SWI) are the most sensitive to demonstrate small and multiple lesions. Any associated DVA and its relationship to the cavernoma should be noted in cases considered for surgical treatment. However, in the acute setting, demonstration of an underlying cavernoma within a parenchymal haemorrhage is usually impossible, including differentiating a brainstem cavernoma from hypertensive brainstem/pontine ICH.

Regardless, in all situations in the emergency setting wherein the ICH potentially requires surgical intervention, the questions are:

In this particular case, is urgent vascular imaging essential?

What are the appropriate radiological investigations and what are the pitfalls of selecting inadequate imaging modality?

Once urgent surgical treatment is decided, the extent of preoperative investigations depends upon the speed of deterioration and current condition. The consideration to obtain an angiogram (DSA) is complex and should be decided on an individual basis: a CTA may miss a small AVM or may be unable to differentiate between dilated arterialised veins from a DAVF and an AVM with potential grave consequences from surgery.

Step 2: Urgent Intervention

Frequently, rupture of an AVM results in a small- or moderate-sized intra-parenchymal haemorrhage or SAH. A DAVF with CVR typically causes a parenchymal or ASDH and most haemorrhages from cavernomas are low-volume haematomas. In the absence of a large ICH, these need supportive care and prevention of any aggravating factors. The resulting neurological deficits may need rehabilitation. Acute intervention would only be directed to the VL if the risk of early re-bleeding is deemed high (detailed in the section on definitive intervention). Acute hydrocephalus due to IVH or ICH obstructing cerebrospinal fluid (CSF) pathways would need urgent insertion of an external ventricular drain (EVD).

Reasons for urgent and early intervention are:

(1) decompression or evacuation of ICH causing, or with the potential to cause, clinically significant mass effect due to raised ICP;
(2) CSF drainage for acute hydrocephalus;
(3) in order to prevent re-bleeding from VLs associated with higher risk of early re-bleeding; and
(4) as a relative indication, and in selected cases, the presence of the ICH may technically facilitate the surgical intervention to deal with the underlying VL – 'window of opportunity'.

Those presenting with a large ICH (or ASDH) face either surgical treatment or no active intervention. The main factors to consider are:

(1) Size/volume of the ICH

Small ICHs can be well tolerated without evacuation, while ICH volumes >50 cc^3 are likely to be associated with poor outcome whatever the intervention. The degree of mass effect such as midline shift as a marker of raised ICP influences decision-making: a large ICH exerts a lesser mass effect in patients with underlying brain atrophy.

(2) Location of the ICH

Deep locations or those occupying eloquent areas are less favourable for surgical evacuation due to a higher chance of post-intervention lasting neurological deficits. Larger haematomas presenting near the cortical surface or in a lobar location are more technically favourable than a similar size clot in a deep or eloquent location. A small ICH obstructing CSF pathways can result in obstructive hydrocephalus.

(3) Age

Older patients have a limited capacity to recover, particularly in the presence of significant comorbidity.

(4) GCS

Alert or slightly drowsy patients (GCS 13–15) would not usually require surgical evacuation of the ICH. Exceptions are described in sections on intervention. Patients with a poor motor score (e.g. abnormal flexion or extension to painful stimuli) are more likely to have a poor outcome: invasive evacuation may be deemed futile.

(5) The rate of deterioration

The prognosis of those with gradual deterioration is possibly better than those with abrupt deterioration. The reasons of further deterioration may be due to ICH expansion, surrounding swelling, or development of hydrocephalus. Surgical evacuation may be more readily considered in those who deteriorated later rather than those who presented in extreme condition, due to a severe primary insult, from the onset.

These factors influence the decision of whether to observe or intervene. As further significant deterioration is likely to be associated with irreversible neurological damage, in many cases, the decision to intervene should be prompt.

A decision not to intervene may be based on advanced age, prior expression of wishes by patients, or a devastating clinical condition (e.g. abnormal posturing, dilated pupils), unsurmountable pre-morbidity, or imaging appearance indicating the futility of surgery.

The characteristics of the ICH or ASDH dictate the initial management, which is directed towards (Figure 1)

(1) ameliorating the effects of increased ICP;
(2) addressing potential aggravating factors detrimental to neurological outcome; and
(3) addressing potential factors leading to expansion of the haematoma, including re-bleeding and anticipating the development of hydrocephalus.

In order to avoid impaired cerebral blood flow and hypoxia consequential to raised ICP, intubation should be considered unless deemed inappropriate due to futility, comorbidities, and advanced age. Mannitol or hypertonic saline administration may facilitate control of elevated ICP. Blood pressure levels should support adequate cerebral perfusion and extreme hypertension should be treated.

Factors aggravating the derangements of cerebral metabolism such as hyperglycaemia or hyponatraemia should be identified and corrected. Early seizures

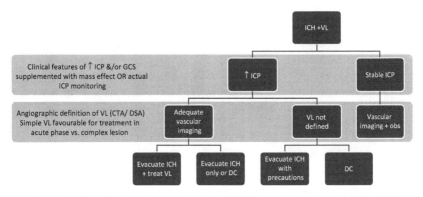

Figure 1 Algorithm for management of ICH with an associated VL. DC, decompressive craniectomy.

will have potential negative effect and despite no conclusive scientific evidence, prophylactic anti-convulsants may be considered.

A) Supratentorial

Considering the factors detailed earlier, in most cases, beneficial surgical interventions for evacuation of the ICH are undertaken on moderate-sized ICH in a superficial location in younger patients with GCS 6–12 (flexing or localising to pain or obeying commands with relatively large ICH). For some deep or eloquent haematomas, a decompressive craniectomy (DC) without evacuation of the ICH is considered. In the presence of an underlying VL, especially if not completely evaluated or complex, DC rather than direct evacuation of the ICH is the safer option (Figure 2). In older patients, hypertension or amyloid angiopathy are more common aetiologies where the threshold for active invasive intervention is much lower.

B) Infratentorial

Infratentorial VLs include AVMs, tentorial DAVF, and cavernomas, the latter are often located in the brainstem. In addition to the considerations in managing supratentorial haemorrhages, as described earlier, the compactness of posterior fossa results in a propensity for early obstructive hydrocephalus due to obstruction around the aqueduct or fourth ventricle. Hence urgent intervention is directed to address the hydrocephalus or the mass effect of the ICH or both. A possible workflow previously described for spontaneous cerebellar haematomas without identifiable VLs can be applied to these cases but with precautions given the underlying VL (Figure 3).[5]

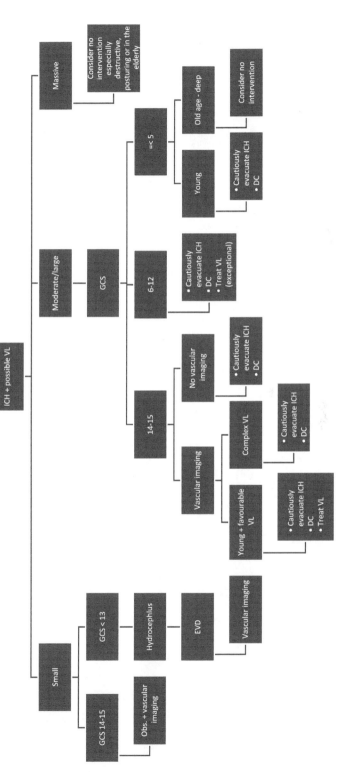

Figure 2 Algorithm for management of supratentorial ICH with a suspected associated VL.

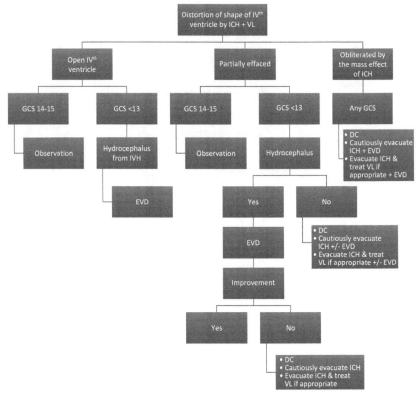

Figure 3 Algorithm for management of infratentorial ICH
with an associated VL.

Considerations, Modifications, and Precautions in the Management of ICH Requiring Surgical Intervention without Tackling the Underlying Lesion

If urgency in dealing with ICH precludes further radiological investigations to avoid delay, is it acceptable to proceed without? And what precautions or modifications of the acute intervention is needed?

In these circumstances, the plan involves adequate control of ICP resulting from the mass effect of the ICH or ASDH without disturbing the underlying VL, which may be too complex to tackle in the acute conditions or has not been adequately defined or investigated yet to allow safe direct surgical management. The first consideration is whether it is feasible to access the ICH to allow decompression through a trajectory that does not involve the VL or confer added injury to the uninvolved functional neural structures. If these are not achievable, then consider performing a DC instead. However, the configuration of the craniectomy should allow access to the VL in the event of future surgical exploration. When evacuating a haematoma, caution should be exercised by undertaking partial evacuation, aiming to avoid disturbance of the underlying VL. A partial haematoma evacuation can be supplemented with a DC when necessary. At times, unexpected bleeding from a VL may occur. This may necessitate proximal vascular control to rescue the situation.

Considerations, Modifications and Precautions in Surgical Intervention of ICH Concomitant with Treatment of the Underlying Lesion

See later.

Step 3: Definitive Intervention in the Acute Phase

After addressing any mass effect from the intracranial haemorrhage, the management of the underlying VL (provided it was adequately evaluated by appropriate investigations) must be considered. This can be:

(1) Concomitant with evacuation of the mass-producing intracranial haematoma:

    (a) if technically favourable in appropriately selected conditions;
    (b) if associated with a high risk of early re-bleeding, or
    (c) if unplanned.

(2) Soon after evacuation of the intracranial haematoma:

    (a) if associated with a high risk of early re-bleeding and appropriate for endovascular treatment;
    (b) if associated with a high risk of early re-bleeding but was not fully evaluated at the time of the initial procedure; or
    (c) if associated with a high risk of early re-bleeding but conditions were inappropriate to proceed with concomitant intervention prior to stabilisation of the clinical condition.

(3) Soon before evacuation of the mass-producing intracranial haematoma:

    (a) if associated with a high risk of early re-bleeding and appropriate for endovascular treatment with a safe time window prior to evacuation of the intracranial haematoma.

(4) Sometimes the early endovascular treatment of an underlying VL is appropriate (e.g. high risk of further haemorrhage), even if the ICH does not require evacuation.

Endovascular and surgical treatments are complimentary and should be considered by the team. Factors that are considered are shown in Table 1.

The angio-architectural characteristics of AVMs that increase the risk of haemorrhage include associated flow or intranidal aneurysms, deep venous drainage, venous outflow compromise, and deep or specific locations such as the cerebellum.[2,3,6] Associated flow or intranidal aneurysms may be the source of the bleeding and hence may carry an increased risk of re-bleeding. Aneurysms associated with AVMs may be classified into those that are at usual locations found in about 3–4% of the adult population (Type I), those that are flow related on a proximal segment of an arterial feeder (Type II) or more distally on the feeder to the nidus beyond the last branching (Type III), or finally an intranidal aneurysm (Type IV).[7] An intranidal aneurysm is probably associated with an increased risk of early re-bleeding.

The factors increasing the difficulties and potential adverse outcomes from surgery are best assessed by the grading systems of Spetzler–Martin, Spetzler–Ponce, and Lawton–Young. The Spetzler–Martin grade is calculated by adding the points given for the nidus size (1 for <3 cm, 2 for 3–6 cm, and 3 for >6 cm), pattern of venous drainage (0 superficial and 1 for deep), and eloquence (0 non-eloquent and 1 for eloquent). The Lawton–Young classification added factors such as age, haemorrhagic classification, perforator supply, and the configuration of the nidus being either compact or diffuse. The factors that increase the difficulties and potential adverse outcomes from surgery include a large-sized nidus, deep and eloquent locations that not only include cortical location but also white matter tracts involvement, age, and a less compact nidus.

Stereotactic radiosurgery (SRS) is often used to treat an AVM following patient recovery after a haemorrhage. The nidus must receive an adequate radiation dose while minimising collateral damage by use of a steep dose gradient. A nidus >3 cm in diameter is less favourable for a single-fraction SRS. There is an interval delay often of 3–4 years until the AVM is obliterated after treatment, during which the risk of haemorrhage continues. Therefore, SRS is less favourable for AVMs with a higher risk of re-bleeding in the short term. On some occasions, the associated flow aneurysm regresses following obliteration of the AVM.

Factors favourable for endovascular embolisation are solitary or few arterial feeders that are amenable for endovascular access. However, even in well-selected cases, curative rates are mostly modest. Furthermore, this intervention often requires multiple sittings, each carrying risks of complication.

Table 1 Correlating risk factors and surgical considerations with urgency of intervention for different VLs.

	Risk factors	Surgical considerations	Urgent surgical intervention	Urgent endovascular intervention
AVM	Aneurysm Deep location Previous haemorrhage Venous outflow compromise	Avoid premature venous compromise	Evacuate ICH only or DC ICH evacuation + AVM resection in very selected cases	Ruptured flow related or intranidal aneurysm
DAVF	CVR Borden type III + Cognard types III + IV Venous ectasia Previous haemorrhage Location	Accurate localisation and disconnection of CVR Locations not readily amenable to endovascular	If higher risk of early re-bleeding	If higher risk of early re-bleeding
Cavernoma	Previous haemorrhage Location Genetic type CCM3 (cerebral cavernous malformations 3)	Preserve DVA	Very rare	Nil

Elimination of the future risk of haemorrhage is only achieved by total extirpation of the AVM. Partial treatments may in fact worsen the prognosis.[2,3,6]

In DAVF, the clinical presentation, course, and the risk of bleeding depend upon the underlying pathophysiology, which is venous hypertension and its magnitude. The Cognard or Borden classifications are based on the pattern of venous outflow and direction and the involvement of the sinuses or sinus wall.

The risk of haemorrhage reaches 40–65% for Borden type III and Cognard types III and IV.[3] However, the hallmark of aggressive presentation with haemorrhage is seen when the DAVF involves CVR due to venous hypertension. The indications for treatment are severe symptoms, haemorrhage, or harbouring factors associated with high risk of haemorrhage. The latter include: (i) cortical venous drainage, which is by far the most important risk factor with an annual bleeding risk of 4–11%, especially if symptomatic; (ii) location in the anterior cranial fossa or at the tentorial incisura; (iii) retrograde sinus flow; and (iv) venous ectasia/venous varix, with an annual bleeding risk of 10–50%.

The intracranial haemorrhage associated with DAVF, given that its origin is from the arterialised bridging and surface cortical veins, is commonly ICH with possible associated SAH or IVH and SDH. These are not only associated with a 30% mortality, but the increased re-bleeding rate can be as high as 35% in 2 weeks, dictating early intervention following presentation with a haemorrhage.

For cavernomas, the risk of haemorrhage per lesion that has never clinically presented with bleeding is extremely small, being 0.5%/year risk of bleeding.[4] The risk of subsequent haemorrhage after a haemorrhagic presentation is slightly increased to 3%/year and decreasing by time, with higher values in males and the brainstem. By far, most haemorrhages are of low volume with minimum consequences apart from perhaps a brainstem location.

A) Indications and Timing for Intervention for AVM in the Presence of an ICH

Step 1: Establish the Origin of Bleeding Whether from the AVM Nidus or from an Associated Related Aneurysm

The distribution of the haemorrhage or the location of the ICH may indicate the source of rupture (Figure 4). However, this may be uncertain, particularly in the presence of a flow aneurysm.

In clear cut cases, with absence of a significant ICH, endovascular obliteration of the aneurysm or even proximal occlusion of the arterial feeder in the absence of *en passage* branches should be undertaken. It is somewhat controversial whether these flow aneurysms carry a high risk of re-bleeding in the short term: early endovascular selective obliteration of the aneurysm may be

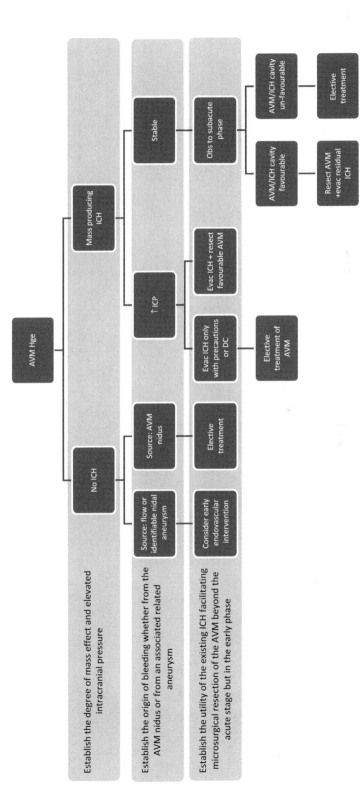

Figure 4 Algorithm for management of ruptured AVM in the acute phase.

undertaken in this situation, even if a delayed AVM resection is planned. This is especially the case when the origin of the haemorrhage is uncertain and/or the general condition require a period of time for stabilisation prior to definitive delayed surgery.

If the flow aneurysm is accessible during early surgery (either to evacuate the ICH and/or resect the AVM), then it can be clipped during the primary procedure.[7]

In some complex AVMs, especially those with recurrent haemorrhage, selective endovascular occlusion or partial obliteration of the relevant part of the nidus is a reasonable option if a prominent intranidal aneurysm is identified as a potential source of the bleeding.

Step 2: Establish the Degree of Mass Effect and Elevated Intracranial Pressure

In the absence of a mass-producing ICH, it is preferable to treat the AVM electively, in a clinically stable patient, to optimise obliteration and recovery rates. If there is hydrocephalus, an EVD is inserted and elective AVM treatment conducted later. In many cases, a moderately large supratentorial ICH can be tolerated, and if in doubt it is reasonable to monitor the ICP initially. If ICP is elevated, evacuation of the ICH alone is appropriate, taking precautions to avoid the AVM or restricting surgery to a DC. Nevertheless, for well-defined and favourable lesions, consider evacuation of the ICH and resection of the AVM concomitantly.

Step 3: Establish the Utility of the Existing ICH Facilitating Microsurgical Resection of the AVM beyond the Acute Stage but in the Early Phase

Although the risk of re-bleeding from an AVM is elevated within the first year or two, very early re-bleeds rarely occur. However, in stable patients, early AVM resection beyond the acute phase (first 48 hours) may be considered due to the presence of the ICH providing a corridor of access and thereby a 'window of opportunity'. Although technical difficulties including the adherence of the AVM to the acute clot can be detrimental, in the subacute phase (5 days to 3 weeks), the ICH liquefies. The potential concern regarding worse definition of the nidus in the presence of the ICH has been reported not to be an issue in the subacute phase, with very good obliteration rates.[8,9] The good clinical outcome and acceptable persistent neurological deficits after surgery mitigated against the presumed negative influence of not waiting for deficit recovery.

Surgical planning for AVM resection in the presence of an ICH utilises approaches to the nidus via the ICH cavity after localisation of the main arterial feeders. It is essential to obtain a preoperative angiogram to characterise the anatomy. A preoperative CTA (or MRI) demonstrates the relationship of the location of the AVM to the ICH cavity. Although resection of an AVM concomitantly with evacuation of an acute ICH is not normally recommended, small surgically favourable AVMs can be resected. Adopting this strategy of operating to resect the AVM in the subacute stage has reported some good results, even in lesions of higher Spetzler grades[9] where the corridor of access facilitates access to deep locations.

Nuances of AVM Surgery in the Presence of an ICH

The presence of a mass-producing ICH necessitates certain precautions:

- The craniotomy should be of sufficient size to provide adequate exposure of both the AVM and the ICH. The initial step involves identification of the draining veins and feeders. This requires careful dissection at regions of friable brain adjacent to the ICH with extra care to protect the draining veins at the initial stages. In the acute phase, the clot adherent to the nidus poses difficulties in defining the edge of the nidus, increasing the propensity of tearing the vessels during the dissection. However, the liquifying haematoma when operating in the subacute stage after the haemorrhage facilitates this step.
- In the presence of an ICH, during access to the nidus, avoid premature exposure of the nidus via the ICH before access to the main feeders and consider partial ICH evacuation to access the deep feeders. During dissection of the nidus, make use of the adjacent ICH to protect eloquent white matter tracts and cortex.
- Two patterns are encountered: in one, the AVM nidus is located superficial to an ICH cavity; while in the other, the AVM is located deep to the ICH. For a superficial AVM, use a trans-sulcal approach, avoiding eloquent brain where possible. Use the draining vein to guide access; complete a full dissection of the superficial part of the nidus first. Then utilise the deep ICH cavity for deep definition of the nidus. If there is urgent need for intra-operative decompression as a first step, perform partial evacuation of ICH in the beginning. For a deeply located AVM, utilise the ICH cavity for access to the nidus. For complex AVMs, avoid premature exposure of the nidus before access to the main arterial feeders. Again, it must be emphasised to protect the main superficial draining veins and the trajectory should avoid eloquent cortex.

Special Considerations for Management of ICH Complicating Endovascular Intervention

Managing an ICH due to AVM rupture provoked during an endovascular procedure can be most challenging. Usually this occurs in the context of planned staged endovascular embolisation of a complex AVM. In cases with a large ICH that definitely requires surgery, it is imperative to evaluate and study the imaging directly with interventional radiologist prior to any procedure. The main reason for the intraprocedural haemorrhage is premature compromise of the venous outflow by the embolic material or by thrombosis. As such, the intranidal pressure is high. Tackling such an AVM directly during a surgical procedure at the time of ICH evacuation can result in massive haemorrhage that cannot be controlled until the AVM is completely resected. In addition, there may be associated disproportional brain swelling due to the venous hypertension, adding to the difficulty of the procedure.

The first step is to establish from the interventionalist the volume of the nidus that is occluded by embolisation and identify the regions of residual filling. In selected cases, AVM resection with the ICH evacuation may be considered if the majority of the nidus has been embolised. There is still potentially increased intranidal pressure and microsurgical access to the deep surface of the nidus is not easy given the non-compressible nature of embolic materials. Furthermore, active haemorrhage may be observed amongst the embolic material in the seemingly occluded segments that is not amenable for haemostasis until the whole AVM is extirpated.

If a partially embolised AVM with an ICH necessitates surgery, a partial evacuation, avoiding the nidus, or a DC is preferred. Release of the tamponade effect may result in significant haemorrhage: the surgeon and anaesthetist should be prepared for this, and if feasible, the procedure should be performed with a second experienced surgeon and the wisdom of an interventional radiologist in the operating room.

In all these cases, ensure that any anticoagulation measures used during the embolisation procedure have been adequately reversed.

B) Indications and Timing for Intervention for DAVF in the Presence of an ICH or ASDH

Intracranial DAVF presents with intracranial haemorrhage due to venous hypertension with CVR. The A-V fistula within the dura may be adjacent to the wall of a venous sinus and involves a bridging vein or occasionally multiple bridging veins that become arterialised with reflux into cortical veins. As such, the re-bleeding rate is high and can occur early, with a rate as high as 35% within 2 weeks. Therefore, regardless of the magnitude of haemorrhage, early intervention to obliterate the DAVF after haemorrhage should be considered.

Urgent Endovascular Treatment of DAVF Presenting with Haemorrhage

The flow chart (Figure 5) indicates the timing of endovascular or possible surgical treatment with different degrees of intracranial haemorrhage, including the need for ICH or ASDH evacuation.

Nuances of DAVF Surgery, Especially in the Presence of an ICH or ASDH

In any situation, surgical treatment of an intracranial DAVF requires sufficient preoperative imaging that almost certainly includes a CTA and a DSA.

The principal concept of surgery for DAVF involves intradural localisation of the responsible arterialised bridging vein(s) at the site of the dural fistula and disconnecting it by clipping or coagulation and dividing it as close as possible as it emanates from the dura at the site of the DAVF.[3,10] In most cases, this is technically straightforward once the fistula is accurately localised. Erroneous early obliteration of a draining vein of an AVM wrongly thought to be a DAVF will result in detrimental consequences.

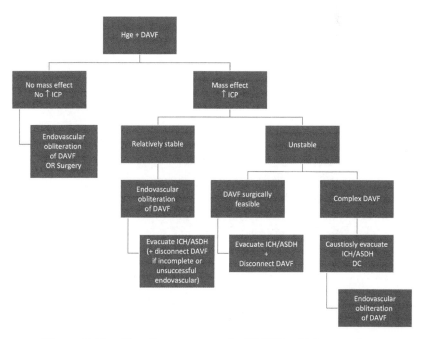

Figure 5 Algorithm for management of DAVF with haemorrhage in the acute phase.

Evacuation of a large ASDH provides the space to access and disconnect the DAVF, especially in locations such as adjacent to the superior sagittal sinus (SSS), parafalcine, or middle fossa along the sphenoparietal sinus. During evacuation of the ASDH, avoid tearing any of the arterialised bridging or cortical veins as these may bleed profusely. After evacuation of a large medial frontal ICH, access to the anterior fossa is enhanced where a typically ethmoidal type DAVF involves an arterialised vein providing CVR adjacent to the crista galli.

Surgical difficulties may be encountered as a result of brain swelling, precluding safe access to deeply located DAVFs such as the petrosal type or those along the tentorial hiatus, which require a supracerebellar approach. Patience together with general measures to achieve brain relaxation including CSF retrieval and drainage aim to avoid excessive retraction.

Some DAVFs harbour multiple transosseos vascular channels through the skull. In these cases, potentially significant blood loss may be encountered by merely performing a craniotomy. Anticipation and anaesthetic preparation for this situation together with rapid sequential haemostasis may salvage the consequences.

C) Indications and Timing for Intervention for Cavernomas in the Presence of an ICH

Rarely, a large mass-producing ICH is the result of an underlying cavernoma. Unless the existence of a cavernoma is already known, identification of a cavernoma on imaging of a large ICH is almost impossible. In these cases, given that a small lesion such as a cavernoma would be in the midst of the ICH, in most cases, it is resected together with the ICH evacuation. One important consideration is to be aware of the possible associated coexistence of an important DVA. These developmental anomalies frequently provide venous drainage to normal regions and their disruption may result in venous infarctions. They are associated with the nonfamilial cavernomas and are not the source of haemorrhage. Identification of such a DVA may not be at all easy in the presence of a large acute ICH. The added value of having a preoperative angiogram is not to confuse a DVA with other VLs.

Most peri- or extra-lesional ICHs from cavernomas are small and do not require any intervention. Depending on location and accessibility of the cavernomas as well as the recovery of deficits (if any), those presenting with haemorrhage, in particular multiple episodes, are considered for elective resection.

Timing for Intervention for Brainstem Cavernomas

Cavernomas located in the brainstem require special consideration due to the proximity to highly eloquent neural structures. Even minor degrees of haemorrhage may be associated with significant neurological deficit. Due to this fact, recurrent haemorrhages are more readily detected and probably cavernomas in these locations have a true propensity for increased re-bleeding rates.[4] Many of these episodes occur in clusters with possible long periods free from haemorrhage. Factors such as the extent of neurological deficits and their recovery, age, and exact location, including proximity to an accessible pial surface, influence treatment strategies. Pitfalls in estimating proximity to a pial surface occur in the presence of an acute haematoma: once the haematoma resolves, it may become apparent that the cavernoma is deep and surrounded by functional neural tissue. Some MRI sequences overestimate the extent of the lesion 'blooming artefact'. Exophytic lesions are most technically favourable although require great care during dissection of the deep surface.

Although the deficits from a brainstem haemorrhage can be devastating, the haematoma does not usually require urgent intervention. If there is obstructive hydrocephalus, insertion of an EVD is needed. Severe bulbar dysfunction may require early intubation, subsequent tracheostomy, and/or gastrostomy. Only rarely, in the event of progressive deterioration, is urgent surgical decompression required.

Due to the bleeding recurrence rate, surgery should be considered as a management option. Controversy exists whether treatment is required following one, two, or more proven clinical episodes of haemorrhage. The decision may vary according to whether the cavernoma is superficial or deep. The next controversy is whether to resect early after a first haemorrhage or electively at a later stage (see Table 2). Again, the associated DVA must be preserved.

Clinical Scenarios Highlighting Initial Evaluation and Management Pathways

Based on the algorithms described in the previous text, this section covers:

- examples of which ICH are suspected to be due to a VL
- examples of ICH needing immediate intervention without full investigations and technical pitfall avoidance during the emergency surgical management
- examples demonstrating selection and timing of intervention in fully investigated ICH in the acute setting.

Table 2 The timing of surgery for brainstem cavernomas, including the advantages and disadvantages of early intervention.

	Pros	**Cons**
Early surgery after haemorrhage	• The associated haematoma brings the lesion towards the surface and provides an access corridor to the cavernoma. • Performing surgery while neurological deficit exists but temporarily stabilised allows the underlying problem to be dealt with and permits rehabilitation and recovery rather than subjecting the patient to potential further setback from surgery after recovering the deficits. • Minimises the potential for re-bleeding	• Cavernoma within the clot may be ill-defined and associated with increased chance of residual cavernoma. • The reported 'no added new deficit' may camouflage iatrogenic neural injury as there was no chance to assess natural reversibility of presenting deficit. • Even if the haematoma seemingly extends to the surface on imaging, it may in fact contain a small rim or intermingled with functional neural tissue which becomes vulnerable to injury through the trajectory
Elective delayed surgery after haemorrhage	• The presence of a surrounding gliotic membrane formed especially after multiple haemorrhages somewhat protect deep and surrounding neural tissue from circumferential dissection and define the limits of the cavernoma. • Imaging following resolution of the haemorrhage better defines the extent and actual location of the cavernoma to plan the safe corridor. • Allows recovery of any deficits from haemorrhage	• Risk of recurrent cluster haemorrhage • May lose the opportunity to take advantage of the existing haematoma providing surgical access to the cavernoma

Supratentorial Haematomas: Different Case Scenarios

1. A 56-year-old male patient with a history of hypertension presented with acute headache. On examination, he was E3, V4, M6 with a left homonymous hemianopia. There was no motor weakness.

Despite the history of hypertension and lobar ICH, this is not a typical location for a 'hypertensive' ICH (Figure 6). The cone-shaped extension into the lateral ventricle makes an underlying AVM a possibility. Hence, full evaluation requires a DSA, whether or not a CTA was performed. This is particularly helpful in the event of any future deterioration.

The clinical condition including the GCS coupled with the minimal mass effect of the ICH do not dictate urgent need for ICH evacuation. Given the size of the ICH, there is a possibility of development of added surrounding swelling, necessitating surgery later.

2. A 72-year-old female with no prior clinical history presented with collapse, E3 V4 with no comprehension to obey commands.

Despite the size of the ICH, there is modest mass effect, highlighting underlying cerebral atrophy (Figure 7). Even if there is an underlying VL, given the

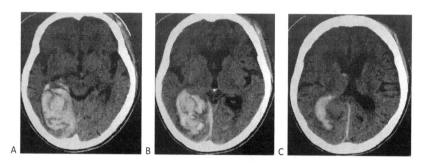

Figure 6 Non-contrast CT head demonstrating right ICH and IVH.

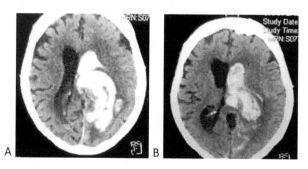

Figure 7 Non-contrast CT head demonstrating left ICH with IVH.

deep location, direct surgery acutely on the ICH and VL is not required. There is potential for deterioration due to hydrocephalus that would warrant consideration of an EVD. It is reasonable with this ICH to defer angiography until clinically stable, especially with the current irritability that may require intubation just to complete the investigation.

3. A 42-year-old male collapsed after complaining of severe headaches and there were no witnessed seizures. There was no eye opening or verbal response, and he was flexing to pain with evident right hemiparesis (E1, V1, M3).

A CTA performed at the time of the CT scan showed an AVM on the deep aspect of the large ICH occupying most of the centrum semiovale (Figure 8). Following the scan, the left pupil was slightly larger. The deep location of the probable AVM favours partial evacuation of the ICH to control the mass effect. Despite a seemingly small AVM, the temptation to tackle the AVM without having an angiogram should be resisted. Not only is the CTA not enough to define the VL, any feeding arteries and draining veins are deep and will not be readily exposed from the trajectory used to evacuate the ICH. Once the patient reasonably recovers after the acute intervention, an angiogram will guide future management options.

4. A 53-year-old presented with acute headaches, partial visual field defect, and grade 3/5 left hemiparesis, with the upper limb more affected than the lower limb.

There is a moderately large ICH on the CT scan. The CTA and DSA confirm a small AVM subcortical nidus fed by distal M4 segment of the precentral branch of MCA and an early draining cortical vein to the SSS (Figure 9). Liquefaction of the haematoma between days 5 and 21 provide an optimal window to

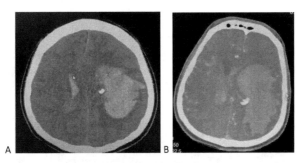

Figure 8 (A) Contrast-enhanced CT and (B) CTA demonstrating left ICH and IVH resultant of ruptured AVM.

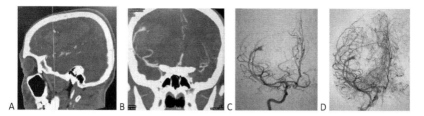

Figure 9 Sagittal (A) and coronal (B) CTA and DSA (C, D) demonstrating right ICH secondary to ruptured small AVM.

facilitate microsurgical resection of the AVM. Alternatively, waiting longer to permit clinical recovery and elective treatment of the AVM is reasonable. Although this is not technically challenging, the alternative option is SRS but this does not protect against the risk of re-bleeding in the first 2–3 years wherein the risk of recurrent haemorrhage is elevated. In this case, whenever there is deterioration in the acute phase, a craniotomy to evacuate the ICH and resection of the AVM at the same time using the techniques described earlier is feasible and advantageous.

5. A 61-year-old female presented with acute headaches. In the first 6 hours she was confused. She subsequently still complained of headaches but otherwise had a GCS of 15 points and no neurological deficits.

The head CT scan showed a parenchymal ICH in the medio-orbital left frontal lobe extending from the anterior fossa (Figure 10A–D). The angiogram with ICA and ECA injections demonstrated filling of an 'ethmoidal' type DAVF with the dural arterial feeders from the anterior ethmoidal branches of the ophthalmic artery entering the anterior fossa and involving a cortical arterialised vein draining towards the anterior SSS, with multiple venous pouches (Figure 10E, 10F). The coronal reconstruction showed the dilated dural arterial branches on the right with CVR and the cortical arterialised vein emerging intradurally adjacent to the left aspect of the crista galli with a venous varix (Figure 10G). This is a Cognard type IV DAVF. The neuro-interventionalist considered that the vascular access was not ideal for effective endovascular embolisation. As these have a high risk of early re-bleeding and despite the ICH not being large enough to require surgical intervention, an early bifrontal craniotomy, inter-hemispheric approach, and disconnection of the cortical arterialised vein 'flush' with the dura at the skull base after evacuation of the ICH is indicated.

6. A 24-year-old male complained of headaches and multiple generalised seizures.

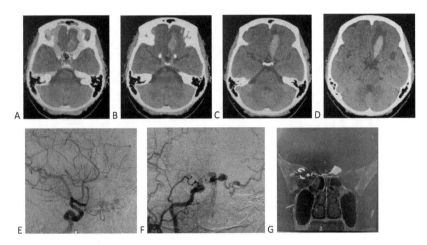

Figure 10 (A, B, C, D, E, F, G) Non-contrast CT head (A–D) demonstrating left basal frontal ICH secondary to DAVF demonstrated on DSA with ICA (E) and ECA (F) injection and coronal CTA (G) showing the location of the VL and venous ectasia.

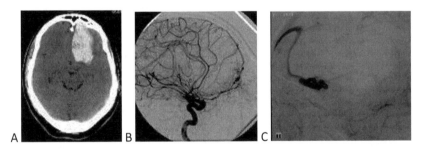

Figure 11 Non-contrast CT head (A) and DSA (B, C) showing left frontal ICH and an AVM nidus draining into the SSS.

The head CT scan showed a relatively large left frontal ICH in more or less a similar location as case 5 (Figure 11A). The patient required intubation and ventilation and was loaded with anticonvulsants. As the basal cisterns were not effaced on the scan and the midline shift was modest, the patient was stable enough to undergo an angiogram, which showed a small AVM at the orbital surface of the frontal pole fed by a prominent fronto-orbital branch of the anterior cerebral artery and draining via a dilated cortical vein towards the SSS (Figure 11B, 11C). On reduction of sedation, the patient did not promptly regain consciousness, and given the substantial size of the ICH a craniotomy, evacuation of the ICH and excision of the AVM was performed.

Cases 5 and 6 highlight the value of obtaining an angiogram to define and dictate the management of the VL.

Infratentorial Haematomas: Different Case Scenarios

1. A 12-year-old boy complained of headaches in the playground at school, on arrival to hospital, he was vomiting repeatedly, with a GCS of 8 (E1, V2, M5).

The CT scan performed after intubation showed a cerebellar ICH extending into both hemispheres, blood in the fourth ventricle, and dilated temporal horns (Figure 12A). An EVD was inserted and an angiogram obtained. This showed a cerebellar AVM with a diffuse nidus fed by the distal cortical branches of the posterior inferior cerebellar artery (PICA) (Figure 12B). Venous drainage was deep, to the straight sinus. The PICA was prominent from its origin and there was a flow aneurysm at the tonsillar loop just beyond the tonsillo-telovelar segment. In this case, given the proximity of the flow aneurysm to the nidus and the presence of a parenchymal ICH and IVH, it cannot be determined with certainty whether the flow aneurysm or the AVM was the source of haemorrhage. A reasonable plan was to endovascularly obliterate the flow aneurysm, allow the patient to recover and be extubated, and once stable, undergo microsurgical resection of the AVM. If performed within 2–3 weeks, the resolving ICH would assist in easier localisation of the nidus. However, endovascular access to the aneurysm through the PICA loops proved difficult and was aborted due to the risks of medullary branch and perforator compromise. Therefore, both the flow aneurysm and the AVM were treated at the same time through a suboccipital posterior fossa craniotomy within few days.

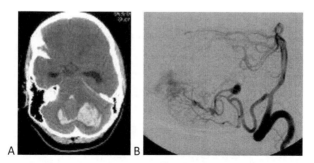

Figure 12 Non-contrast CT head (A) and DSA (B) demonstrating posterior fossa ICH and IVH in the fourth ventricle and a cerebellar AVM with a flow aneurysm on the PICA feeder.

2. A 67-year-old female presented with severe headaches and vomiting. She was drowsy, opening eyes to speech, confused, and unable to stand or walk.

The CT scan and CTA showed a midline vermian cerebellar ICH extending into and obliterating the fourth ventricle (Figure 13A). She underwent an angiogram that revealed an AVM with a nidus of about 3.5 cm fed by distal superior cerebellar artery branches (Figure 13B, 13C). The AVM was located on the left superior cerebellar tentorial surface and drained via the superior petrosal vein to the transverse sinus. Three hours after the angiogram, the patient became unconscious with no eye opening or speech and was flexing to pain (E1, V1, M4). An urgent posterior fossa decompression and possible partial evacuation of the ICH with insertion of an EVD was indicated. The question of whether or not to resect the AVM at the same time depends largely upon the expertise of the available surgeon and the condition of the patient.

3. A 28-year-old female presented with sudden diplopia and left partial ptosis that slightly worsened over 2 days. There was gait imbalance with evidence of impaired proprioception on walking.

A CT scan showed a well-defined hyperdense central midbrain lesion and the MRI showed signal changes in the lesion and perilesional area located in the tegmentum of the midbrain in a left paramedian position, with a fluid level consistent with an intralesional subacute haemorrhage (Figure 14). This is consistent with a cavernoma. The patient should be assessed for any evidence of bulbar dysfunction and commence rehabilitation. This is a first haemorrhagic episode of a deep-seated cavernoma without extension to an accessible pial surface (proximity to surface in the midline of the interpeduncular cistern does not render it surgically favourable).

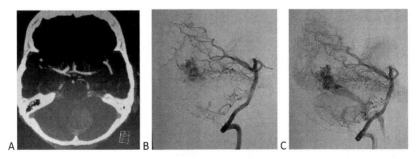

Figure 13 Non-contrast CT head (A) and DSA (B, C) showing a posterior fossa ICH secondary to ruptured AVM fed by distal branches of the SCA.

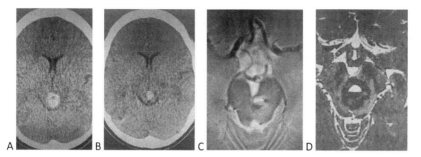

Figure 14 Non-contrast CT head (A, B) demonstrates a well hyperdense lesion and a T2-weighted MRI head (C, D) confirms haemorrhage with a fluid level within the lesion.

4. A 42-year-old male with a known diagnosis of an incidentally found midbrain cavernoma that was untreated after counselling regarding the benefit: risk of surgery collapsed and rapidly deteriorated to extending to pain with anisocoria and irregular breathing.

The head CT scan with sagittal reconstruction shows extensive haemorrhage throughout the brainstem and extending into the diencephalon (Figure 15A). The previous sagittal T1-weighted MRI with gadolinium and the axial T2-weighted images shows the midbrain cavernoma (Figure 15B, 15C). Although it is most uncommon for haemorrhage from cavernomas to be extensive, surgical intervention at this stage is futile.

Step 4: Aftercare

Those with depressed GCS at presentation associated with haemorrhage that require surgery for mass effect require monitoring and management of ICP management in the intensive care unit. Blood pressure control and occasional induced controlled hypotension is required, particularly after resection of a complex AVM and in those when the final haemostasis was achieved with difficulty, blood pressure control is important to avoid normal pressure breakthrough or to minimise the risk of postoperative haemorrhage until remodelling of arterial feeders is achieved.[11]

Any other potential postsurgical complications such as brain swelling, epilepsy, re-bleeding, or postoperative haematomas, and endovascular complications including delayed venous thrombosis or retained catheters require individualised management.

A post-treatment angiogram should be obtained whenever the general and neurological condition allows to ensure obliteration of the treated VL. Planning

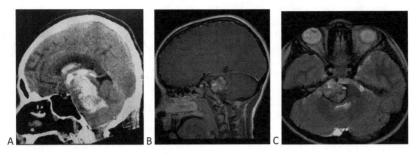

Figure 15 Non-contrast CT head (A) showing extensive brain stem haemorrhage from a previously demonstrated midbrain cavernoma on the MRI (T1-weighted (B) and T2-weighted (C)).

of other treatments including SRS or staged endovascular intervention for specific lesions that have not been surgically excised at this stage, should be considered. Rehabilitation is an important part of managing sequelae.

Conclusion

Managing a patient with a spontaneous intracranial haemorrhage due to a non-aneurysmal vascular abnormality may require prompt complex decision-making. This requires understanding the underlying pathology, natural history, pathophysiology, and the associated risk factors for the underlying VL together with specific considerations for the ICH. The appropriate workup should be targeted to the individual case and include awareness of possible diagnostic pitfalls. The management options may be guided by algorithms but should consider the timely management of mass effect and considered management of any causative VL. Some lesions require specific technical nuances and appreciation of the technical precautions. Appropriate after care should be followed.

References

1. Unterberg AW, Orakcioglu B (2019). Spontaneous Intracranial Haematoma. In Kirollos RW, Helmy A, Thomson S, Hutchinson PJ, eds., *Oxford Textbook of Neurological Surgery*, 1st ed.; Oxford: Oxford University Press, pp. 643–649.
2. Weerakkody RA, Trivedi R, Santarius T, Kirollos RW (2009). Intracranial Arteriovenous Malformations. *British Journal of Neurosurgery*, **21**, 1–5.
3. Morgan M (2019). Arteriovenous Malformation and Dural Arteriovenous Fistulae. In Kirollos RW, Helmy A, Thomson S, Hutchinson PJ, eds., *Oxford Textbook of Neurological Surgery*, 1st ed.; Oxford: Oxford University Press, pp. 591–613.
4. Patel H, Beijnum J (2019). Cavernoma and Angiographically Occult Lesions. In Kirollos RW, Helmy A, Thomson S, Hutchinson PJ, eds., *Oxford Textbook of Neurological Surgery*, 1st ed.; Oxford: Oxford University Press, pp. 651–657.
5. Kirollos RW, Tyagi AK, Ross SA, van Hille PT, Marks PV (2001). Management of Spontaneous Cerebellar Haematomas: A Prospective Treatment Protocol. *Neurosurgery*, **49**(6), 1378–1386.
6. Trivedi R, Kirollos R, Whitfield P (2009). Considerations in the Management of Cerebral Arterio-venous Malformations. *Advances in Clinical Neuroscience and Rehabilitation*, **9**(3), 26–29.
7. Budohoski KP, Mohan M, Millar Z, et al. (2021). Longitudinal Changes in Size of Conservatively Managed Flow-Related Aneurysms Associated with Brain Arteriovenous Malformations. *World Neurosurgery*, **154**, e754–e761.
8. Marcus H, Weerakkody RA, Trivedi R, Santarius T, Kirollos R (2010). Management of Arteriovenous Malformations (AVMs) Presenting with Intracranial Haemorrhage: The Role of Subacute Resection. *British Journal of Neurosurgery*, **24**(1), 95.
9. Barone DG, Marcus HJ, Guilfoyle MR, et al. (2017). Clinical Experience and Results of Microsurgical Resection of Arteriovenous Malformation in the Presence of Space-Occupying Intracerebral Hematoma. *Neurosurgery*, **81**(1), 75–86.
10. Al-Mahfoudh R, Kirollos R, Mitchell P, et al. (2015). Surgical Disconnection of the Cortical Venous Reflux for High-Grade Intracranial Dural Arteriovenous Fistulas. *World Neurosurgery*, **83**(4), 652–656.
11. Morgan MK, Guilfoyle M, Kirollos R, Heller GZ (2019). Remodeling of the Feeding Arterial System after Surgery for Resection of Brain Arteriovenous Malformations: An Observational Study. *Neurosurgery*, **84**(1), 84–94.

Cambridge Elements ≡

Emergency Neurosurgery

Nihal Gurusinghe
Lancashire Teaching Hospital NHS Trust

Professor Nihal Gurusinghe is a Consultant Neurosurgeon at the Lancashire Teaching Hospitals NHS Trust. He is on the Executive Council of the Society of British Neurological Surgeons as the Lead for NICE (National Institute for Health and Care Excellence) guidelines relating to neurosurgical practice. He is also an examiner for the UK and International FRCS examinations in Neurosurgery.

Peter Hutchinson
University of Cambridge, Society of British Neurological Surgeons and Royal College of Surgeons of England

Peter Hutchinson BSc MBBS FFSEM FRCS(SN) PhD FMedSci is Professor of Neurosurgery and Head of the Division of Academic Neurosurgery at the University of Cambridge, and Honorary Consultant Neurosurgeon at Addenbrooke's Hospital. He is Director of Clinical Research at the Royal College of Surgeons of England and Meetings Secretary of the Society of British Neurological Surgeons.

Ioannis Fouyas
Royal College of Surgeons of Edinburgh

Ioannis Fouyas is a Consultant Neurosurgeon in Edinburgh. His clinical interests focus on the treatment of complex cerebrovascular and skull base pathologies. His academic endeavours concentrate in the field of cerebrovascular pathophysiology. His passion is technical surgical training, fulfilled in collaboration with the Royal College of Surgeons of Edinburgh. Finally, he pursues Undergraduate Neuroscience teaching, with a particular focus on functional Neuroanatomy.

Naomi Slator
North Bristol NHS Trust

Naomi Slator FRCS (SN) is a Consultant Spinal Neurosurgeon based at North Bristol NHS Trust. She has a specialist interest in Complex Spine alongside Cranial and Spinal Trauma. She completed her neurosurgical training in Birmingham and a six-month Fellowship in CSF and Trauma (2019). She then went on to complete her Spinal Fellowship in Leeds (2020) before moving to the southwest to take up her consultant post.

Ian Kamaly-Asl
Royal Manchester Children's Hospital

Ian Kamaly-Asl is a full time paediatric neurosurgeon and Honorary Chair at Royal Manchester Children's Hospital. He trained in North Western Deanery with fellowships at Boston Children's Hospital and Sick Kids in Toronto. Ian is a member of council of The Royal College of Surgeons of England and The SBNS where he is lead for mentoring and tackling oppressive behaviours.

Peter Whitfield

University Hospitals Plymouth NHS Trust

Professor Peter Whitfield is a Consultant Neurosurgeon at the South West Neurosurgical Centre, University Hospitals Plymouth NHS Trust. His clinical interests include vascular neurosurgery, neuro oncology and trauma. He has held many roles in postgraduate neurosurgical education and is President of the Society of British Neurological Surgeons. Peter has published widely, and is passionate about education, training and the promotion of clinical research.

About the Series

Elements in Emergency Neurosurgery is intended for trainees and practitioners in Neurosurgery and Emergency Medicine as well as allied specialties all over the world. Authored by international experts, this series provides core knowledge, common clinical pathways and recommendations on the management of acute conditions of the brain and spine.

Cambridge Elements ᐧ

Emergency Neurosurgery

Elements in the Series

Printed in the United States
by Baker & Taylor Publisher Services